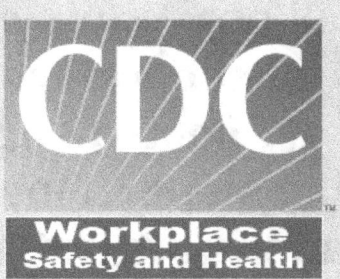

Exposure to Flour Dust and Sensitization Among Bakery Employees

Elena H. Page, MD, MPH
Chad H. Dowell, MS, CIH
Charles A. Mueller, MS
Raymond E. Biagini, PhD

Health Hazard Evaluation Report
HETA 2005–0248–3077
Sara Lee Bakery
Sacramento, California
January 2009

DEPARTMENT OF HEALTH AND HUMAN SERVICES
Centers for Disease Control and Prevention

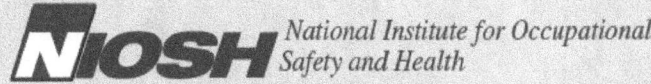
National Institute for Occupational Safety and Health

The employer shall post a copy of this report for a period of 30 calendar days at or near the workplace(s) of affected employees. The employer shall take steps to insure that the posted determinations are not altered, defaced, or covered by other material during such period. [37 FR 23640, November 7, 1972, as amended at 45 FR 2653, January 14, 1980].

CONTENTS

ABBREVIATIONS

ACGIH®	American Conference of Governmental Industrial Hygienists
AIHA	American Industrial Hygiene Association
BAA	Bakery-associated antigens
CalOSHA	California Occupational Safety and Health Administration
CDC	Centers for Disease Control and Prevention
FDA	Food and Drug Administration
GA	General area
GM	Geometric mean
HEPA	High-efficiency particulate air
HHE	Health hazard evaluation
IgE	Immunoglobulin E
IOM	Institute of Occupational Medicine
kU/L	Killiunits per liter of serum
MDC	Minimum detectable concentration
mg/m^3	Milligrams per cubic meter
mL	Milliliter
MQC	Minimum quantifiable concentration
95% CI	95% confidence interval
NAICS	North American Industry Classification System
ND	Nondetectable
NIOSH	National Institute for Occupational Safety and Health
OEL	Occupational exposure limit
OSHA	Occupational Safety and Health Administration
PBZ	Personal breathing zone
PEL	Permissible exposure limit
PR	Prevalence ratio
REL	Recommended exposure limit
STEL	Short-term exposure limit
TLV®	Threshold limit value
TWA	Time-weighted average
WEEL	Workplace environmental exposure level

HIGHLIGHTS OF THE NIOSH HEALTH HAZARD EVALUATION

The National Institute for Occupational Safety and Health (NIOSH) received a confidential employee request for a health hazard evaluation at the Sara Lee Bakery in Sacramento, California. The requestors were concerned about rashes, possibly from exposure to propylene glycol which had been used in the refrigeration system for approximately the past three years. There were concerns with the adequacy of the ventilation system and respiratory symptoms among workers. NIOSH investigators conducted three site visits between August 2005 and March 2006.

What NIOSH Did

- We looked at the operations and work practices in the bakery.

- We looked at the use of propylene glycol in the facility.

- We talked to employees about potential work-related health problems.

- We measured airborne flour dust, α-amylase, and wheat in the bread and bun production departments, office, and distribution areas. We also took measurements during maintenance and sanitation.

- We asked employees to fill out questionnaires about their work and medical history, and health problems they had at work.

- We drew blood from employees and tested it to see if they were sensitized to flour dust, α-amylase, wheat, and certain common allergens.

- We categorized employees into two groups so we could compare symptom and sensitization prevalences between the groups: those with jobs that had higher potential exposure to flour dust and other baking ingredients and those with jobs that had lower potential exposure to these products.

What NIOSH Found

- Propylene glycol did not pose a health risk because it was used in a closed system with little possibility of employee exposure.

- Employees handling unbaked dough or dry ingredients were overexposed to flour dust.

- Employees in the higher-exposure group had significantly higher prevalences of work-related wheezing, runny nose, stuffy nose, and frequent sneezing than employees in the lower-exposure group.

- Employees in the higher-exposure group had a significantly higher prevalence of rash on their face, neck, hands, or arms in the month prior to the survey than employees in the lower-exposure group.

- Employees with current or past jobs in the higher-exposure group were also more likely to be sensitized to wheat.

What Managers Can Do

- Use local exhaust or general ventilation to lower dust levels in the bakery.

- Require use of a vacuum or wet wash method to clean up powder. Do not allow use of compressed air for cleaning.

- Require employees who work with unbaked dough or dry ingredients to wear a respirator until ventilation controls can reduce dust levels.

- Hire a physician to evaluate employees for respiratory and skin symptoms before they begin work and periodically while they handle unbaked dough or dry ingredients.

What Employees Can Do

- Properly wear the respirators provided by the company.

- Report possible work-related health problems to your supervisor so you can be referred for a medical evaluation.

- Use slow, smooth movements when handling powdered ingredients to keep dust levels low.

- Use a vacuum or wet wash method to clean up powder. Do not use compressed air for cleaning.

SUMMARY

NIOSH investigators evaluated dust exposures, rashes, respiratory symptoms, and sensitization to BAA among employees at the Sara Lee Bakery in Sacramento, California. Employees handling unbaked dough or dry ingredients exceeded the CalOSHA PEL and ACGIH TLV for exposure to inhalable flour dust. Employees categorized as having higher potential exposure to flour dust had significantly higher prevalences of work-related wheezing, runny nose, stuffy nose, and frequent sneezing than employees with lower potential exposure. They also had a significantly higher prevalence of rash on their face, neck, hands, or arms in the month prior to the study. We found evidence of both non-specific irritant and allergic upper and lower respiratory symptoms among employees with current and/or past exposure to BAA. Recommendations to reduce flour and allergen exposures are included in this report.

In May 2005, NIOSH received a confidential employee request for an HHE at the Sara Lee Bakery in Sacramento, California. The request concerned rashes, respiratory symptoms, and problems with ventilation and indoor environmental quality. In an August 2005 work site visit we met with management and union representatives, toured the plant, and held confidential medical interviews with employees. We observed potential exposure to flour dust and BAA and received reports of employees with work-related hand dermatitis, cough, eye irritation, and aggravation of pre-existing asthma. We also learned of at least one employee who was diagnosed with baker's asthma.

We returned to the bakery in March 2006. All bakery employees were asked to participate in an evaluation designed to compare sensitization and symptom prevalences between groups categorized as having higher and lower potential exposure to BAA and to more accurately characterize exposure in the different bakery departments. PBZ and GA air monitoring was performed to measure inhalable flour dust and total dust. The inhalable flour dust samples were further analyzed for α-amylase and wheat. The study included a questionnaire, and blood tests for total IgE; IgE specific to flour dust, wheat, and α-amylase; and for a variety of common aeroallergens.

Of 186 bakery employees present during our site visit, 161 (87%) completed the questionnaire. Of these, 96 allowed their blood to be drawn. We observed the process in the bakery and also used information in the scientific literature to assign "lower-exposure" and "higher-exposure" categories to participants. Participants were assigned to either a lower-exposure group or a higher-exposure group based upon their job title at the time of the survey.

We collected 83 PBZ and 19 GA air measurements for inhalable flour dust in the bread and bun production, distribution, engineering, and sanitation departments; and the office and plant management areas. The inhalable flour dust concentrations for PBZ and GA samples for certain job titles in the lower-exposure group had a GM of 0.235 mg/m³, a median of 0.245 mg/m³, with a range between ND (less than 0.12 mg/m³, based on an average sample volume) and 1.4 mg/m³. Of the 23 PBZ measurements for employees in this group, 8 reached or exceeded the CalOSHA PEL and ACGIH TLV of 0.5 mg/m³ TWA for inhalable flour dust. The inhalable flour dust concentrations for PBZ and GA samples in the higher-exposure group had a GM of 3.01 mg/m³, a median of 2.75 mg/m³, with a range between trace (between 0.12 and 0.42 mg/m³, based on an average sample volume) and 65 mg/m³. Of the 60 PBZ measurements for employees in this group, 56 reached or exceeded the CalOSHA PEL and ACGIH TLV for inhalable flour dust.

Employees in the higher-exposure group had a significantly higher prevalence of work-related wheezing than those in the lower-exposure group (14.8% vs. 1.1%). They also had significantly higher prevalences of work-related runny nose, stuffy nose, and frequent sneezing. The higher-exposure group had a significantly higher prevalence of rash on their face, neck, hands, or arms in the month prior to the study.

The prevalences of IgE specific to wheat, inhalable flour dust, and α-amylase were higher in the higher-exposure group at both the ≥ 0.10 kU/L and the ≥ 0.35 kU/L cutoffs, but the differences were not statistically significant. The prevalence of IgE specific to wheat was significantly higher among employees who reported either a current or past job in the higher-exposure group or in production at another bakery at both the ≥ 0.10 kU/L and the ≥ 0.35 kU/L cutoffs, and to flour dust and α-amylase at the ≥ 0.10 kU/L cutoff, compared to the lower-exposure group.

The prevalences of work-related wheezing were 3–5 times higher in employees sensitized to wheat than those who were not sensitized. This difference was statistically significant at the ≥ 0.10 kU/L cutoff for IgE but was not significant at the ≥ 0.35 kU/L cutoff. The prevalences of work-related runny nose was significantly higher among those sensitized to wheat at the ≥ 0.35 kU/L cutoff, but not at the ≥ 0.10 kU/L cutoff. We found no statistically significant differences in work-related symptom prevalences between those above and below the cutoffs for sensitization to α-amylase. Work-related runny nose was significantly more prevalent among those sensitized to flour than those who were not sensitized at the ≥ 0.35 kU/L cutoff, but was not significant at the ≥ 0.10 kU/L cutoff. Atopics (defined by a positive AlaTOP) were significantly more likely to be sensitized to wheat and flour dust at both the ≥ 0.10 kU/L cutoff and ≥ 0.35 kU/L cutoff, and to α-amylase at the ≥ 0.10 kU/L cutoff.

In conclusion, a health hazard exists at the Sara Lee Bakery in Sacramento, California, from exposure to flour dust and other BAA. Recommendations include implementing a variety of engineering and work practice controls, as well as the use of respiratory protection until these controls are implemented. Management should provide a medical surveillance program for employees exposed to BAA.

Keywords: NAICS 311812 (commercial bakeries), flour, inhalable dust, α-amylase, wheat, asthma, rash, respiratory

Introduction

On May 30, 2005, NIOSH received a confidential employee request for an HHE at the Sara Lee Bakery in Sacramento, California. The request stated that employees at the bakery were experiencing rashes, possibly from exposure to propylene glycol, which had been used in the refrigeration system for approximately the past 3 years. The requestors also expressed concerns about the adequacy of the ventilation system, respiratory symptoms among the employees, and indoor environmental quality.

After review of the request and telephone consultations with the employee requestors, Sara Lee's corporate health and safety official, and the plant manager, we made a site visit to the bakery on August 2–3, 2005. The opening conference included the plant manager; the corporate health and safety official; two human resources representatives; and employee representatives of the Bakery, Confection, and Tobacco Union Local 85 and of the International Union of Operating Engineers Local 39. After the conference we toured the facility to observe the operations, work practices, and working conditions. We also interviewed several employees about potential work-related health problems.

We returned to the facility on January 23–25, 2006, to recruit employee volunteers to participate in a more extensive evaluation. On March 25–31, 2006, we conducted industrial hygiene and biological monitoring to characterize employees' exposures and determine the prevalence of sensitization to flour and enzymes, as well as the prevalence of work-related skin and respiratory symptoms.

Process Description

The Sara Lee Bakery in Sacramento, California, is one of approximately 42 bakeries owned and operated by the Sara Lee Bakery Group. It was purchased by Sara Lee from Earthgrains in 2001, but has been operating since 1880, and was originally named Henry Schnatz Bakery. The Sacramento plant makes bread and buns and employs over 200 people in management and administrative positions, sales, transportation, maintenance engineering, and production. The production employees are further divided into those working on the bread and bun lines, in packaging, and in distribution. Approximately 155 production employees and 18 maintenance engineers work at this facility.

Loaf bread is made in the bread line, and hamburger and hot dog buns are made in the bun lines. The plant operates 24 hours a day, 7 days a week, with the bread line operating approximately 120 hours and the bun line operating approximately 130 to 140 hours before shutdown and cleaning. At any one time, approximately 18 employees each work on the bread and the bun lines, including those directly involved with baking, packaging, and distribution. Production employees work staggered 7-hour shifts and receive three 15-minute breaks. The maintenance engineers work 8-hour shifts with six engineers on each shift.

The entire baking process takes approximately 7 hours, and wheat flour is the most frequently handled product. The sponge (a mixture of flour, water, and various additives) is fermented for 3 to 4 hours. Flour is pneumatically added to the sponge in a mixer to produce dough. In some instances, powdered ingredients are manually added to the mixer directly from bags or after being hand-weighed into 5-gallon buckets. Local exhaust ventilation is not used during the manual handling of ingredients. The dough mix is then made into loaves or buns and baked. The baked bread and buns are cut, inspected, bagged, and sent to shipping.

Sanitation is performed on two shifts each week and includes both dry and wet clean-up methods. In the area where dough is mixed, overhead pipes, conveyers, and equipment are blown off with compressed air. Following the removal of dust with the compressed air, the area is dry swept and then scrubbed/hosed down with a mixture of detergents, sanitizers, and water. In other areas of the plant, dry cleaning techniques are used including blowing off equipment with compressed air and dry sweeping. A mixture of detergents, sanitizers, and water are then used for wet cleaning; however, they are only applied as needed to smaller, localized areas.

On the initial site visit, we observed that bakery employees were exposed to flour dust and other allergens including enzymes and spices. Several employees reported hand dermatitis, and at least one had been diagnosed with baker's asthma. Employees also reported aggravation of pre-existing asthma, cough, and eye irritation. No exposure assessment had been done in the past several years. We determined that propylene glycol did not pose a hazard because it was used in an enclosed system with little opportunity for exposure to production employees. We believe that propylene glycol was not responsible for employee symptoms and that these symptoms were likely due to other exposures at the facility.

Based on our initial findings, we decided to further evaluate the respiratory and dermal concerns mentioned in the HHE request, specifically baker's asthma and baker's dermatitis. Wheat and other cereal flours are the main causes of baker's allergy, but other common BAA include enzymatic dough improvers such as fungal α-amylase. Allergic symptoms can develop after months to years, and the risk of developing symptoms increases with increased exposure. Bakers can also experience mucous membrane and respiratory irritation, possibly more commonly than allergic symptoms [Houba et al. 1998]. Baker's dermatitis can result from exposure to wet dough, flours with additives, spices, water, and detergents. Baker's asthma and baker's dermatitis are discussed in greater detail in Appendix A.

During the week of March 25–31, 2006, all employees at the bakery were asked to participate in our evaluation, which was designed to compare sensitization and symptom prevalences between groups of employees with differing levels of exposure to BAA and accurately characterize exposure in the different departments of the bakery. We drew samples of participants' blood and tested it for total IgE; for IgE specific to flour dust, wheat, and α-amylase; and for a variety of common aeroallergens to assess atopy. All participants in this evaluation completed a questionnaire. Questions concerned demographics (age, sex, job title, years worked, work department); personal history of allergies, eczema, asthma, and smoking; having upper and/or lower respiratory symptoms at work in the last month (unrelated to a cold or respiratory infection); and whether those symptoms got better on days off work. Symptoms were considered work related if they were present at work and improved on days away from work. Potential study participants were given a consent form to read and sign should they wish to participate in the study. Each study participant was informed in writing of the results of his or her blood tests and what they meant. A detailed discussion of the methods used for this evaluation is available in Appendix B.

PBZ and GA air sampling conducted during this evaluation was designed to characterize employees' overall exposures to BAA. Task-based sampling was not conducted. While tasks were noted, the specific exposure for each task was not identified. Full shift PBZ and GA air measurements for inhalable flour dust and total dust were collected in the bread and bun production, distribution, engineering, and sanitation departments; and the office and plant management areas. While both PBZ and GA samples were taken in multiple work areas, GA samples were primarily taken in areas where exposure was thought to be low (i.e., office areas). No measurements were taken for transportation workers because they do not work in the bakery building, but drive trucks to deliver product to retailers. A detailed discussion of the methods used for this evaluation is available in Appendix B.

Industrial Hygiene

Most powdered ingredients used in the bakery, except flour, are shipped in paper bags and transferred to 20-gallon plastic drums with an internal depth of approximately 25 inches (see Figure 1). Once the powdered ingredients are transferred into the plastic drums, employees must manually transfer the powdered ingredients to a 5-gallon bucket on the scale. We observed many employees leaning forward with their head inside the drum to scoop out the powder near the bottom. In this position, the employee has greater exposure to the airborne flour dust and other BAA.

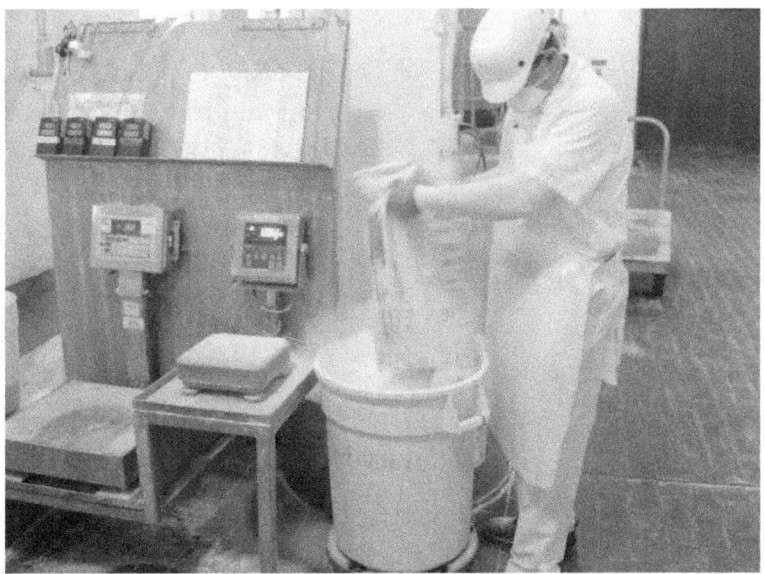

Figure 1. Transfer of powdered ingredient into 20-gallon plastic drum

In the area where bread and bun dough was mixed (the second floor of the bakery) ventilation was limited to general room dilution, primarily used for temperature control. The scales and mixers in this area did not have local exhaust ventilation to reduce exposure to flour dust and other BAA. In the bread and bun loafing and shaping areas (the first floor of the bakery), local exhaust ventilation was limited to areas where flour was applied to the dough, primarily to prevent it from sticking to the machinery. This local exhaust ventilation consisted of exhaust hoods at or directly following the point where flour was applied to the dough. The air collected from the local exhaust hoods was filtered through a dry centrifugal collector with a bag or sock filter and then exhausted back into the plant. Plant engineers did not know the filtration efficiency of the bag or sock filter.

Four employees at the facility were included in a respiratory protection program at the time of our evaluation. Two employees used full-facepiece respirators for pest control activities, and two engineers used half-mask respirators for confined space entry and work in dusty environments. Production employees were not covered by the program and were not required to wear respiratory protection; however, some production employees used dust masks voluntarily. Some of these employees were observed wearing their dust masks incorrectly.

We observed employees using poor handling techniques to weigh and transfer ingredients into the mixer bowls (see Figure 2 and Figure 3). These poor handling techniques included quick, manual transfer of powdered ingredients. The employee dropped the powder from an excessive height into a 5-gallon bucket (used as a scale pan) and into the mixers (both through the opening in the top of the mixer and directly into the mixer bowls). Both of these movements generated a dust cloud in the employee's breathing zone and likely contributed to his high flour dust exposures.

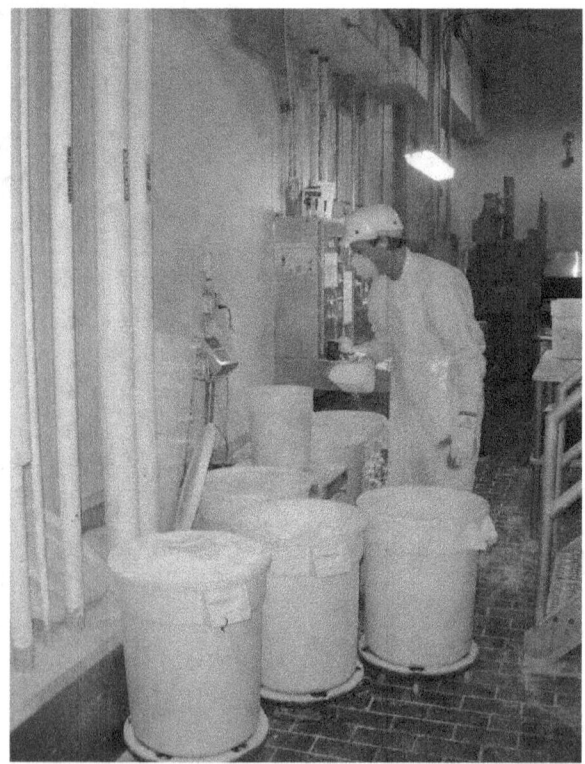

Figure 2. Transfer of powdered ingredient from 20-gallon drum to 5-gallon bucket (scale pan)

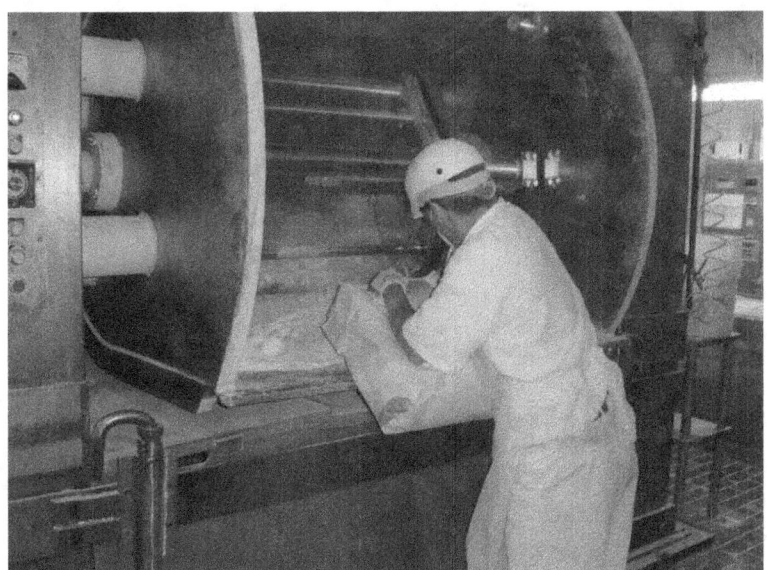

Figure 3. Transfer of powdered ingredient into mixer bowl

We observed the process in the bakery and also used information in the scientific literature to assign "lower-exposure" and "higher-exposure" categories to participants. The lower-exposure group included employees who worked in the office areas (sales, plant management, and administrative employees) and those in production management, transportation, distribution, bread or bun wrap, and oven areas (oven and pan stacker employees). These employees either did not handle the product at all or only handled baked bread or buns, not dough. The higher-exposure group included the remainder of bread and bun production employees and forepersons, sanitation, and engineers. These employees either handled raw ingredients and/or dough or came in contact with the machinery that handled ingredients or dough. Persons who reported prior job assignments at Sara Lee that fell into the higher-exposure group or who had worked in production at another bakery were assigned to the past higher-exposure group.

We collected 83 PBZ and 19 GA air measurements for inhalable flour dust in the bread and bun production, distribution, engineering, and sanitation departments; and the office and plant management areas. The samples were analyzed for α-amylase and wheat. Results are summarized as follows: inhalable flour dust (Table 1), α-amylase (Table 3), and wheat (Table 4). Table 2 identifies the subset of PBZ air measurements for inhalable flour dust that reached or exceeded the CalOSHA PEL. A listing of the individual results is available in Appendix C.

RESULTS AND DISCUSSION
(CONTINUED)

The 36 inhalable flour dust concentrations for PBZ and GA samples for the subset of job titles that were sampled in the lower-exposure group had a GM of 0.235 mg/m³, a median of 0.245 mg/m³, with a range between ND (less than 0.12 mg/m³, based on an average sample volume) and 1.4 mg/m³. Of the 23 PBZ measurements for employees in this group, 8 reached or exceeded the CalOSHA PEL and ACGIH TLV of 0.5 mg/m³ TWA for inhalable flour dust. The 23 PBZ samples from the lower-exposure group had a range of ND to 1.4 mg/m³. The 13 GA samples for the lower-exposure group had a range of ND to 0.49 mg/m³.

The 66 inhalable flour dust concentrations for PBZ and GA samples in the higher-exposure group had a GM of 3.01 mg/m³, a median of 2.75 mg/m³, with a range between trace (between 0.12 and 0.42 mg/m³, based on an average sample volume) and 65 mg/m³. Of the 60 PBZ measurements for employees in this group, 56 reached or exceeded the CalOSHA PEL and ACGIH TLV for inhalable flour dust. The 60 PBZ samples in the higher-exposure group ranged from trace to 65 mg/m³. The six GA samples in the higher-exposure group ranged from trace to 8.2 mg/m³.

Table 1. Personal breathing-zone and area air sampling results for inhalable flour dust

Job title	Number of samples	GM (mg/m³)	Median (mg/m³)	Min (mg/m³)	Max (mg/m³)
Divider	7	3.26	3.40	1.3	6.3
Foreperson (bread and bun)	6	3.71	3.95	2.0	7.3
Jobber	1	1.20	1.20		
Mixer	8	4.00	3.25	1.3	18
Moulder	4	2.16	3.35	*	7.3
Oven	4	0.400	0.445	*	0.55
Pan Line	5	3.40	3.70	0.45	12
Pan Stacker	1	1.20	1.20		
Scaler	3	5.56	7.80	1.1	20
Sponge Mixer	4	25.2	27.5	8.2	65
Utility	1	0.840	0.840		
Wrap	21	0.335	0.250	†	1.4
Unknown (bun)	1	18.0	18.0		
Distribution‡	6	§	§	†	*
Engineering	6	0.594	0.525	*	2.4
Office and plant management	4	¶	¶	†	†
Sanitation‡	20	2.51	1.45	0.55	64

*Trace: between 0.12 and 0.42 mg/m³ (based on an average sample volume)
†ND: less than 0.12 mg/m³ (based on an average sample volume)
‡Includes one foreperson
§None of the samples were above the MQC
¶None of the samples were above the MDC

RESULTS AND DISCUSSION
(CONTINUED)

Table 2. Number of personal breathing-zone samples for inhalable flour dust that reached or exceeded the CalOSHA PEL

Job title	Number of Samples	Number ≥ CalOSHA PEL*	Job title	Number of Samples	Number ≥ CalOSHA PEL*
Divider	6	6	Scaler	2	2
Foreperson[†]	6	6	Sponge Mixer	4	4
Jobber	1	1	Utility	1	1
Mixer	6	6	Wrap	17	5
Moulder	3	3	Unknown (bun)	1	1
Oven	4	2	Distribution[‡]	1	0
Pan Line	4	3	Engineering	6	3
Pan Stacker	1	1	Sanitation[‡]	20	20

*CalOSHA PEL = 0.5 mg/m^3
[†]Bread and bun
[‡]Includes one foreperson

Table 3. Personal breathing-zone and area air sampling results for α-amylase

Job title	Number of samples	GM (ng/m^3)	Median (ng/m^3)	Min (ng/m^3)	Max (ng/m^3)
Divider	7	0.232	0.300	*	0.45
Foreperson (bread and bun)	6	10.8	12.4	1.1	220
Jobber	1	0.120[‡]	0.120[‡]		
Mixer	8	123	237	3.2	11,000
Moulder	4	0.602	0.980	*	1.2
Oven	4	0.0690	0.0845[‡]	*	0.13
Pan Line	5	1.30	1.10	*	8.9
Pan Stacker	1	0.160[‡]	0.160[‡]		
Scaler	3	3.25	4.10	2.0	4.2
Sponge Mixer	4	41.4	35.0	4.4	1,200
Utility	1	0.550	0.550		
Wrap	21	§	§	*	*
Unknown (bun)	1	17.0	17.0		
Distribution[†]	6	§	§	*	*
Engineering	6	0.131[‡]	0.105[‡]	*	0.27
Office and plant management	4	0.221	0.140[‡]	*	1.1
Sanitation[†]	20	1.05	1.03	*	31

*ND: less than 0.18 ng/m^3 (based on an average sample volume)
[†]Includes one foreperson
[‡]Median or GM is less than the MDC (based on an average sample volume)
§None of the samples were above the MDC

We measured total dust concentrations to determine whether they correlated well with the inhalable flour dust. In general, total dust and inhalable dust sample results may differ because inhalable dust samplers are more efficient for collecting large particles. We collected 23 PBZ and 14 GA air measurements for total dust side-by-side with the inhalable flour dust samples. Total dust concentrations ranged from ND (less than 0.12 mg/^{3}) to 30 mg/m^3. Measurements for three employees exceeded the OSHA PEL for particulates not otherwise regulated of

15 mg/m³, and measurements for six employees exceeded the NIOSH REL for grain dust (oat, wheat, and barley) of 4 mg/m³. The logs of the total dust and inhalable flour dust concentrations were significantly, positively correlated (r = 0.94, p < 0.01).

Table 4. Personal breathing-zone and area air sampling results for wheat

Job title	Number of samples	GM (ng/m³)	Median (ng/m³)	Min (ng/m³)	Max (ng/m³)
Divider	7	20,000	16,000	6,700	89,000
Foreperson (bread and bun)	6	20,000	22,500	9,500	36,000
Jobber	1	2,900	2,900		
Mixer	8	16,200	18,500	2,900	69,000
Moulder	4	13,100	29,500	†	150,000
Oven	4	1,420	1,550	780	2,200
Pan Line	5	25,300	29,000	900	320,000
Pan Stacker	1	3,600	3,600		
Scaler	3	9,550	10,000	6,700	13,000
Sponge Mixer	4	90,600	125,000	25,000	180,000
Utility	1	5,700	5,700		
Wrap	21	420	260‡	†	2,600
Unknown (bun)	1	58,000	58,000		
Distribution*	6	§	§	†	†
Engineering	6	1,110	1,060	†	28,000
Office and plant management	4	§	§	†	†
Sanitation*	20	10,500	5,450	1300	900,000

*Includes one foreperson
†ND: less than 300 ng/m³ (based on an average sample volume)
‡Median or GM is less than the MDC (based on an average sample volume)
§None of the samples were above the MDC

We also looked to see if the wheat and α-amylase correlated with the inhalable flour dust concentrations. The logs of wheat (r = 0.93, p < 0.01) and α-amylase (r = 0.64, p < 0.01) were significantly, positively correlated with the logs of the inhalable flour dust concentrations.

Medical

Of 186 employees present in the bakery during the site visit, 161 (87%) completed the questionnaire. Of these, 96 allowed their blood to be drawn. Sixteen employees refused to participate, and nine could not be contacted during the visit.

Demographics

Demographic information for employees is provided in Table 5. Employees showed no difference in mean age between the lower- and higher-exposure groups, and they were similar in sex distribution. Of employees in the higher-exposure group, 15% reported current asthma compared to 6% in the lower-exposure group; however, among persons who had never smoked, the difference was more pronounced (18% of the higher-exposure group compared to 2% of the lower-exposure group). Nobody reported being diagnosed with baker's asthma.

Table 5. Demographic information, by current exposure group

	Higher-exposure group n = 65–66*	Lower-exposure group n = 93–95*
Mean age	44	44
Mean tenure	13 years	16 years
Male	89%	82%
Smoking status		
Never	50%	55%
Former	33%	23%
Current	17%	22%

*Denominators vary due to missing information

Work-Related Symptoms

Employees in the higher-exposure group had higher prevalences of some work-related symptoms than those in the lower-exposure group (see Table 6). This was most striking for work-related wheezing, with 15% of the higher-exposure group reporting work-related wheezing or whistling in the chest compared to 1% of the lower-exposure group (PR = 13 57; CI: 1.76, 104.44). Employees in the higher-exposure group also reported significantly more work-related runny nose, stuffy nose, and frequent sneezing (see Table 6). We also calculated prevalence ratios for work-related cough, wheezing, and shortness of breath while controlling for smoking; and the results were similar. Of the higher-exposure group, 27% reported having a rash on their face, neck, hands, or arms in the month prior to the study, compared to 14% of the lower-exposure group (PR = 1.99; CI: 1.05, 3.78).

Table 6. Prevalence of work-related symptoms, by current exposure group

Work-related symptom	Higher-exposure group n = 61–64* Number (percent)	Lower-exposure group n = 91–93* Number (percent)	Prevalence ratio (95% Confidence Interval)
Cough	8 (13%)	4 (4%)	3.00 (0.99, 11.42)
Wheeze or whistling in chest	9 (15%)	1 (1%)	13.57 (2.27, 174.40)
Unusual shortness of breath	7 (11%)	4 (4%)	2.56 (0.81, 10.68)
Runny nose	10 (16%)	4 (4%)	3.81 (1.25, 11.61)
Stuffy nose	11 (18%)	6 (6%)	2.75 (1.07, 7.05)
Sinus problems	10 (16%)	7 (8%)	2.05 (0.83, 5.11)
Dry or irritated eyes	12 (19%)	10 (11%)	1.78 (0.82, 3.86)
Frequent sneezing	13 (21%)	7 (8%)	2.68 (1.13, 6.34)

*Denominators vary due to missing information

Traditionally, a level ≥ 0.35 kU/L of specific IgE is considered a positive test, which means that the person is sensitized; however, the test we used (IMMULITE 2000) has an FDA-cleared cutoff of 0.10 kU/L IgE. Therefore, we report results at both cutoffs. The prevalences of IgE specific to wheat, flour dust, and α-amylase were higher in the higher-exposure group at both the ≥ 0.10 kU/L and the ≥ 0.35 kU/L cutoffs, but these differences were not statistically significant (see Table 7). A number of employees who had jobs in the lower-exposure group at the time of the site visit reported past work in a higher-exposure group job at Sara Lee or in production at another bakery. The prevalence of IgE specific to wheat was significantly higher among employees who reported either a current or past job in the higher-exposure group or in production at another bakery at both the ≥ 0.10 kU/L and the ≥ 0.35 kU/L cutoffs, and to flour dust and α-amylase at the ≥ 0.10 kU/L cutoff, compared to the lower-exposure group (See Table 8). The prevalences of sensitization to α-amylase and wheat at the ≥ 0.35 kU/L cutoff among the higher-exposure group in this evaluation are similar to those found in other studies, which have demonstrated prevalences of sensitization of 5%–28% to wheat and 2%–16% to α-amylase [Houba et al. 1996]. A NIOSH study of 534 blood donors demonstrated the prevalences of specific IgE to wheat, flour, and α-amylase of 3.6%, 5.8%, and 1.0%, respectively [Biagini et al. 2004]. These are similar to the prevalences of sensitization among the lower-exposure group at the ≥ 0.35 kU/L cutoff (Table 8).

Table 7. Prevalence of sensitization to bakery-associated antigens, by current exposure group

Measure of sensitization	Higher-exposure group n = 45 Number (percent)	Lower-exposure group n = 51 Number (percent)	Prevalence ratio (95% Confidence Interval)
IgE to α-amylase			
≥ 0.10 kU/L	5 (11%)	2 (4%)	2.83 (0.65, 18.84)
≥ 0.35 kU/L	3 (7%)	1 (2%)	3.40 (0.49, 43.25)
IgE to flour			
≥ 0.10 kU/L	19 (42%)	12 (24%)	1.79 (0.98, 3.27)
≥ 0.35 kU/L	9 (20%)	6 (12%)	1.70 (0.66, 4.40)
IgE to wheat			
≥ 0.10 kU/L	16 (36%)	12 (24%)	1.51 (0.80, 2.84)
≥ 0.35 kU/L	12 (27%)	7 (14%)	1.94 (0.84, 4.51)

Table 8. Prevalence of sensitization to bakery-associated antigens, by current and/or past exposure group

Measure of senstization	Higher-exposure group (either current or past) n = 63 Number (percent)	Lower-exposure group n = 33 Number (percent)	Prevalence ratio (95% Confidence Interval)
IgE to α-amylase			
≥ 0.10 kU/L	7 (11%)	0	+inf* (1.02, +inf)
≥ 0.35 kU/L	4 (6%)	0	+inf (0.58, +inf)
IgE to flour			
≥ 0.10 kU/L	26 (41%)	5 (15%)	2.72 (1.15, 6.43)
≥ 0.35 kU/L	13 (21%)	2 (6%)	3.40 (0.82, 14.20)
IgE to wheat			
≥ 0.10 kU/L	23 (37%)	5 (15%)	2.41 (1.01, 5.75)
≥ 0.35 kU/L	17 (27%)	2 (6%)	4.45 (1.09, 18.12)

*Positive infinity or undefined

Relationship Between Sensitization to BAA and Work-Related Symptoms

The prevalences of work-related wheezing were 3–5 times higher in employees sensitized to wheat than those that were not sensitized (see Table 9). The difference was statistically significant at the ≥ 0.10 kU/L cutoff for IgE but was not significant at the ≥ 0.35 kU/L cutoff ($p = 0.06$). The prevalences of work-related runny nose was significantly higher among those sensitized to wheat at the ≥ 0.35 kU/L cutoff, but not at the ≥ 0.10 kU/L cutoff ($p = 0.10$). The prevalences of work-related frequent sneezing were higher among wheat sensitized persons but were not significant ($p = 0.11$ at the ≥ 0.35 kU/L cutoff and 0.09 at the ≥ 0.10 kU/L cutoff).

No statistically significant differences appeared in work-related symptom prevalences between those above and those below the cutoffs for sensitization to α-amylase (see Table 10). Work-related runny nose was significantly more prevalent among those sensitized to flour than those that were not sensitized ($p = 0.03$) at the ≥ 0.35 kU/L cutoff but was not significant at the ≥ 0.10 kU/L cutoff (see Table 11).

Table 9. Prevalence of work-related symptoms among employees sensitized and not sensitized to wheat

Work-related symptoms	IgE to wheat			IgE to wheat		
	< 0.10 kU/L n = 65–67	≥ 0.10 kU/L n = 24–27	p value	< 0.35 kU/L n = 72–75	≥ 0.35 kU/L n = 17–18	p value
Cough	4 (6%)	5 (20%)	0.11	6 (8%)	3 (17%)	0.37
Wheeze or whistling in chest	3 (5%)	6 (25%)	0.01	5 (7%)	4 (24%)	0.06
Unusual shortness of breath	6 (9%)	2 (8%)	1.00	6 (8%)	2 (11%)	0.65
Runny nose	7 (11%)	6 (25%)	0.10	7 (10%)	6 (35%)	0.01
Stuffy nose	10 (15%)	5 (19%)	0.76	11 (15%)	4 (22%)	0.48
Sinus problems	11 (16%)	3 (12%)	0.75	11 (15%)	3 (17%)	1.00
Dry or irritated eyes	11 (17%)	6 (23%)	0.55	13 (18%)	4 (22%)	0.74
Frequent sneezing	10 (15%)	8 (31%)	0.09	12 (16%)	6 (33%)	0.11

Table 10. Prevalence of work-related symptoms among employees sensitized and not sensitized to α-amylase

Work-related symptoms	IgE to α-amylase			IgE to α-amylase		
	< 0.10 kU/L n = 83–86	≥ 0.10 kU/L n = 6–7	p value	< 0.35 kU/L n = 86–89	≥ 0.35 kU/L n = 3–4	p value
Cough	7 (8%)	2 (29%)	0.14	8 (9%)	1 (25%)	0.35
Wheeze or whistling in chest	8 (10%)	1 (17%)	0.48	9 (10%)	0	1.00
Unusual shortness of breath	8 (9%)	0	1.00	8 (9%)	0	1.00
Runny nose	11 (13%)	2 (33%)	0.21	12 (14%)	1 (33%)	0.38
Stuffy nose	14 (16%)	1 (14%)	1.00	15 (17%)	0	1.00
Sinus problems	13 (15%)	1 (14%)	1.00	13 (15%)	1 (25%)	0.49
Dry or irritated eyes	15 (18%)	2 (29%)	0.61	16 (18%)	1 (25%)	0.57
Frequent sneezing	15 (18%)	3 (43%)	0.13	17 (19%)	1 (25%)	1.00

Table 11. Prevalence of work-related symptoms relationship among employees sensitized and not sensitized to flour

Work-related symptoms	IgE to flour			IgE to flour		
	< 0.10 kU/L n = 62–64	≥ 0.10 kU/L n = 27–30	p value	< 0.35 kU/L n = 75–78	≥ 0.35 kU/L n = 14–15	p value
Cough	4 (6%)	5 (18%)	0.13	6 (8%)	3 (20%)	0.16
Wheeze or whistling in chest	4 (6%)	5 (19%)	0.12	6 (8%)	3 (21%)	0.15
Unusual shortness of breath	7 (11%)	1 (4%)	0.43	7 (9%)	1 (7%)	1.00
Runny nose	8 (13%)	5 (19%)	0.52	8 (11%)	5 (36%)	0.03
Stuffy nose	9 (15%)	6 (20%)	0.55	11 (14%)	4 (27%)	0.26
Sinus problems	10 (16%)	4 (14%)	1.00	11 (14%)	3 (20%)	0.69
Dry or irritated eyes	11 (18%)	6 (21%)	0.78	14 (18%)	3 (20%)	1.00
Frequent sneezing	10 (16%)	8 (28%)	0.26	13 (17%)	5 (33%)	0.16

While the lower cutoff appears to be more sensitive at identifying employees who are sensitized, this may be a trade-off for lower specificity. Since we do not have a gold standard to which to compare our results, we cannot determine the true sensitivity or specificity of the tests at either cutoff.

Few symptoms were significantly related to sensitization, and of those that were, no clear pattern of which cutoff was better

Results and Discussion
(CONTINUED)

emerged. The small number of participants in the evaluation may have limited our ability to detect significant differences. In addition, nonallergic work-related irritation symptoms, which are thought to be more common than allergic symptoms among employees exposed to BAA, may have obscured the relationship between sensitization and symptoms because the symptoms due to allergy and those due to irritation are similar.

Atopy is the predisposition toward having allergic diseases. We determined whether employees were atopic by AlaTOP. We found no significant difference in the prevalence of atopy between groups when looking at the AlaTOP (47% [21/45] of the higher-exposure group vs. 41% [21/51] of the lower-exposure group, p = 0.59). Geometric mean total IgE for the higher-exposure group was 49.6 kU/L compared to 40.2 kU/L for the lower-exposure group (p = 0.51). Atopics (defined by a positive AlaTOP) were significantly more likely to be sensitized to wheat and flour at both the ≥ 0.10 kU/L cutoff and ≥ 0.35 kU/L cutoff and to α-amylase at the ≥ 0.10 kU/L cutoff (see Table 12). This is consistent with past studies of bakery-associated allergy.

Table 12. Prevalence of sensitization to bakery-associated antigens, by atopy

AlaTOP	IgE to α-amylase		IgE to flour		IgE to wheat	
	≥ 0.10 kU/L	≥ 0.35 kU/L	≥ 0.10 kU/L	≥ 0.35 kU/L	≥ 0.10 kU/L	≥ 0.35 kU/L
Positive (n = 42)	6 (14%)	3 (7%)	21 (50%)	13 (31%)	21 (50%)	15 (36%)
Negative (n = 54)	1 (2%)	1 (2%)	10 (19%)	2 (4%)	7 (13%)	4 (7%)
p value	0.04	0.32	< 0.01	< 0.01	< 0.01	< 0.01

Conclusion

A health hazard exists at the Sara Lee Bakery in Sacramento, California, from exposure to flour dust and other BAA. Dust levels for employees who handled the unbaked dough or powdered ingredients exceeded the CalOSHA PEL and ACGIH TLV for inhalable flour dust during our evaluation. Some employees' exposures also exceeded the OSHA PEL for particulates not otherwise classified and the NIOSH REL for grain dust. Lack of ventilation controls and poor work practices contributed to high dust exposures.

Employees in the higher-exposure group had significantly higher prevalences of work-related wheezing, runny nose, stuffy nose, and frequent sneezing than employees in the lower-exposure group. They also had a significantly higher prevalence of rash on their face, neck, hands, or arms in the month prior to the study. Employees who reported having a job in the higher-exposure group (either currently or in the past) were significantly more likely to be sensitized to wheat at both cutoff levels considered to be "positive" tests for sensitization, and to flour and α-amylase at the ≥ 0.10 kU/L cutoff. Atopic employees were at higher risk of being sensitized to BAA.

RECOMMENDATIONS

1. Use a semidowndraft ventilation booth while manually weighing and transferring powdered ingredients (see Figure 4). A vertical air shower can push airborne dust out of the employee's breathing zone and into the exhaust hood. Without the air shower, eddy currents can form around the employee and stir up dust. All tasks associated with the manual transfer of powdered ingredients (weighing, scooping, etc.) should be performed inside the booth under the air shower.

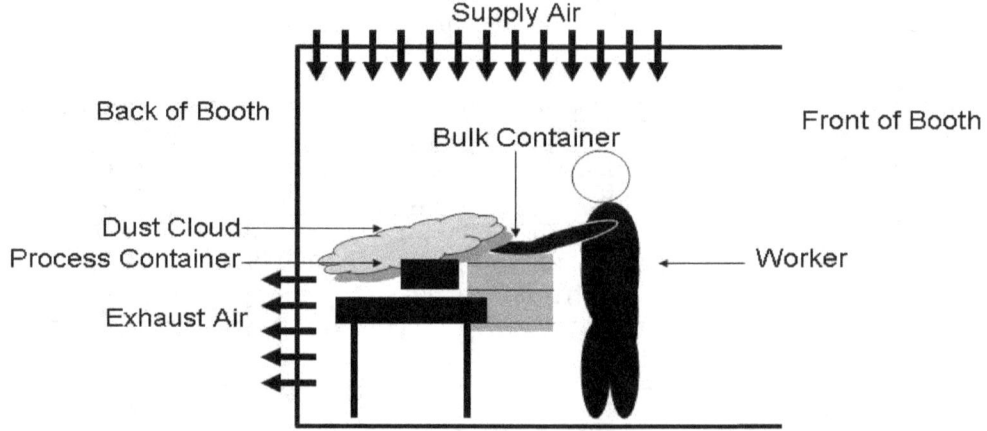

Figure 4. Diagram of semidowndraft ventilation booth

2. Use shorter drums or gravity-fed powder dispensers so employees do not have to reach so far into the drum. Maintaining a space between the employee's face and the top of the drum enables the booth's ventilation to capture the dust before it reaches the employee's breathing zone. Reducing the drum height can reduce employee dust exposures.

3. Train employees to use slow, smooth movements when handling powdered ingredients to keep dust concentrations low. Transport distances between the bulk and process containers should be kept to a minimum. The height at

which powdered ingredients are dropped into a container should also be kept to a minimum. This distance can be reduced by using shallow tubs as scale pans instead of the deeper 5-gallon buckets currently used.

4. Use a pneumatic transfer system equipped with a bag dump station to transfer powdered ingredients from the scaling operation to the mixers. The system should be equipped with a negative pressure bag dump station that captures and exhausts airborne dust out of the employee's breathing zone. This will eliminate the need to add powdered ingredients to the mixers through the opening in the top or directly to the mixing bowl.

5. Use a central dust collection system for all local exhaust capture hoods, or equip the local exhaust capture hoods with filters that effectively remove the particulate. A central dust collection system would allow all dust collected from the various local exhaust hoods to be effectively filtered and exhausted from the facility, preventing the reintroduction of dust into the workplace. If a central exhaust system is not feasible, the filter efficiency on the current local exhaust hoods, which recirculate air into the workplace, should be evaluated to ensure they are effectively removing the dust.

6. Do not use compressed air to clean surfaces. A HEPA vacuum or wet-wash method should be used. A central dust collection system can be used to support sanitation procedures by equipping the system with vacuum attachment points.

7. Require employees to use respiratory protection until engineering controls can be implemented that reduce employee exposure below the CalOSHA PEL and ACGIH TLV for inhalable flour dust. Implementation should follow the OSHA respiratory protection standard [29 CFR 1910.134]. Respiratory protection should be used as a temporary control, not a permanent solution to controlling dust exposures.

Employees working on the second floor of the bakery, all sanitation employees, and pan line employees (on the first floor) should wear a respirator with a minimum assigned protection factor of 50 because of the level of exposure to flour dust. Respirators with an assigned protection factor of 50 include the following:

a. Any air-purifying full facepiece respirator equipped with an N100, R100, or P100 filter
b. Any powered air-purifying respirator equipped with a tight-fitting facepiece (half or full facepiece) and a high-efficiency filter
c. Any negative pressure (demand) supplied-air respirator equipped with a full facepiece
d. Any continuous flow supplied-air respirator equipped with a tight-fitting facepiece (half or full facepiece)
e. Any negative-pressure (demand) self-contained respirator equipped with a full facepiece

Employees working on the first floor, not including pan line employees and distribution employees, should wear a respirator with a minimum assigned protection factor of 10 because of the level of exposure to flour dust. Respirators with an assigned protection of 10 include the following respirators:

a. Any air-purifying elastomeric half-mask respirator equipped with an N100, R100, or P100 particulate filter
b. Appropriate filtering facepiece respirator
c. Any air-purifying full facepiece respirator equipped with an N95, R95, P95, or greater particulate filter
d. Any negative pressure (demand) supplied-air respirator equipped with a half-mask

These respirator recommendations are based on employees' overall exposures for the different departments measured during this HHE and on guidelines presented in the NIOSH Respirator Selection Logic [NIOSH 2004]. Because task-based exposures were not evaluated, we could not identify those tasks that require respiratory protection and those that may not. Additional sampling for inhalable dust should be conducted to identify those specific tasks with exposures that exceed the CalOSHA PEL for inhalable flour dust. For example, dry cleaning with compressed air may require respiratory protection while wet cleaning with a mop may not. In addition, employees' PBZ exposures should be reevaluated following the implementation of engineering controls (i.e., ventilation changes) that could decrease exposures. Once task-based exposures are determined, the NIOSH Respirator Selection Logic should be followed

RECOMMENDATIONS
(CONTINUED)

to ensure that the correct level of respiratory protection is selected. Either of these sampling efforts could reduce the number of employees required to be in the respiratory protection program.

8. Institute a medical surveillance program for employees who are exposed to flour dust. At a minimum, use a medical questionnaire that focuses on skin, mucous membrane, and respiratory symptoms that are work related. The questionnaire should be given prior to placement in a job with flour exposure, and periodically thereafter. In addition, employees should report work-related skin, eye, and respiratory symptoms to their supervisor. Employees who report work-related symptoms should be evaluated by a physician experienced in occupational medicine or allergy. If employees develop occupational rhinitis or asthma, they should be removed from exposure to flour and placed in a job without flour exposure while maintaining their earnings, seniority, and other rights and benefits.

REFERENCES

Biagini RE, MacKenzie BA, Sammons DL, Smith JP, Striley CA, Robertson SK, Snawder JE [2004]. Evaluation of the prevalence of anti-wheat, anti-flour dust, and anti-α-amylase specific IgE antibodies in US blood donors. Ann Allergy Asthma Immun 92:649–653.

CFR. Code of Federal Regulations. Washington, DC: U.S. Government Printing Office, Office of the Federal Register.

Houba R, Heederick D, Doekes G, van Run P [1996]. Exposure sensitization relationship for α-amylase allergens in the baking industry. Am J Respir Crit Care Med 154:130–136.

Houba R, Doekes G, Heederick D [1998]. Occupational respiratory allergy in bakery workers: a review of the literature. Am J Ind Med 34(6):529–546.

NIOSH [2004]. NIOSH respirator selection logic. Cincinnati, OH: U.S. Department of Health and Human Services, Centers for Disease Control and Prevention, National Institute for Occupational Safety and Health, DHHS (NIOSH) Publication No. 2005-100. [www.cdc.gov/niosh/docs/2005-100/]. Date accessed: Janaury 2009.

In evaluating the hazards posed by workplace exposures, NIOSH investigators use both mandatory (legally enforceable) and recommended OELs for chemical, physical, and biological agents as a guide for making recommendations. OELs have been developed by Federal agencies and safety and health organizations to prevent the occurrence of adverse health effects from workplace exposures. Generally, OELs suggest levels of exposure to which most employees may be exposed up to 10 hours per day, 40 hours per week for a working lifetime without experiencing adverse health effects. However, not all employees will be protected from adverse health effects even if their exposures are maintained below these levels. A small percentage may experience adverse health effects because of individual susceptibility, a pre-existing medical condition, and/or a hypersensitivity (allergy). In addition, some hazardous substances may act in combination with other workplace exposures, the general environment, or with medications or personal habits of the employee to produce health effects even if the occupational exposures are controlled at the level set by the exposure limit. Also, some substances can be absorbed by direct contact with the skin and mucous membranes in addition to being inhaled, which contributes to the individual's overall exposure.

Most OELs are expressed as a TWA exposure. A TWA refers to the average exposure during a normal 8- to 10-hour workday. Some chemical substances and physical agents have recommended STEL or ceiling values where health effects are caused by exposures over a short period. Unless otherwise noted, the STEL is a 15-minute TWA exposure that should not be exceeded at any time during a workday, and the ceiling limit is an exposure that should not be exceeded at any time.

In the U.S , OELs have been established by Federal agencies, professional organizations, state and local governments, and other entities. Some OELs are legally enforceable limits, while others are recommendations. The U.S. Department of Labor OSHA PELs (29 CFR 1910 [general industry]; 29 CFR 1926 [construction industry]; and 29 CFR 1917 [maritime industry]) are legal limits enforceable in workplaces covered under the Occupational Safety and Health Act. NIOSH RELs are recommendations based on a critical review of the scientific and technical information available on a given hazard and the adequacy of methods to identify and control the hazard. NIOSH RELs can be found in the *NIOSH Pocket Guide to Chemical Hazards* [NIOSH 2005]. NIOSH also recommends different types of risk management practices (e.g., engineering controls, safe work practices, employee education/training, personal protective equipment, and exposure and medical monitoring) to minimize the risk of exposure and adverse health effects from these hazards. Other OELs that are commonly used and cited in the U.S. include the TLVs recommended by ACGIH, a professional organization, and the WEELs recommended by the American Industrial Hygiene Association, another professional organization. The TLVs and WEELs are developed by committee members of these associations from a review of the published, peer-reviewed literature. They are not consensus standards. ACGIH TLVs are considered voluntary exposure guidelines for use by industrial hygienists and others trained in this discipline "to assist in the control of health hazards" [ACGIH 2007]. WEELs have been established for some chemicals "when no other legal or authoritative limits exist" [AIHA 2007].

Outside the U.S., OELs have been established by various agencies and organizations and include both legal and recommended limits. Since 2006, the Berufsgenossenschaftliches Institut für Arbeitsschutz (German Institute for Occupational Safety and Health) has maintained a database of international

OELs from European Union member states, Canada (Québec), Japan, Switzerland, and the U.S. [www.hvbg.de/e/bia/gestis/limit_values/index.html]. The database contains international limits for over 1250 hazardous substances and is updated annually.

Employers should understand that not all hazardous chemicals have specific OSHA PELs, and for some agents the legally enforceable and recommended limits may not reflect current health-based information. However, an employer is still required by OSHA to protect its employees from hazards even in the absence of a specific OSHA PEL. OSHA requires an employer to furnish employees a place of employment free from recognized hazards that cause or are likely to cause death or serious physical harm [Occupational Safety and Health Act of 1970 (Public Law 91–596, sec. 5(a)(1))]. Thus, NIOSH investigators encourage employers to make use of other OELs when making risk assessment and risk management decisions to best protect the health of their employees. NIOSH investigators also encourage the use of the traditional hierarchy of controls approach to eliminate or minimize identified workplace hazards. This includes, in order of preference, the use of: (1) substitution or elimination of the hazardous agent, (2) engineering controls (e.g., local exhaust ventilation, process enclosure, dilution ventilation), (3) administrative controls (e.g., limiting time of exposure, employee training, work practice changes, medical surveillance), and (4) personal protective equipment (e.g., respiratory protection, gloves, eye protection, hearing protection). Control banding, a qualitative risk assessment and risk management tool, is a complementary approach to protecting employee health that focuses resources on exposure controls by describing how a risk needs to be managed [www.cdc.gov/niosh/topics/ctrlbanding/]. This approach can be applied in situations where OELs have not been established or can be used to supplement the OELs, when available.

Federal OSHA considers flour dust as general nuisance dust (particulates not otherwise regulated); therefore the PEL is 15 mg/m^3. The CalOSHA PEL and ACGIH TLV for inhalable flour dust are 0.5 mg/m^3. British Columbia, Ontario, Hong Kong, and Ireland also have occupational exposure limits for inhalable flour dust of 0.5 mg/m^3. No occupational exposure limits specific for α-amylase or wheat have been developed. The NIOSH REL for grain dust (oat, wheat, and barley) is 4 mg/m^3.

Baker's Asthma

Baker's asthma is one of the most common forms of occupational asthma. Ramazinni was the first to describe baker's asthma in 1700. Case reports from the beginning of the 20th century established it as an allergic disease because of the observed combination of positive skin tests to flour extracts and respiratory symptoms suggestive of asthma [Brisman 2002]. Despite the fact that the risks of exposure to bakery dust have been known for centuries, the incidence of baker's asthma appears to be steadily increasing [Houba et al. 1998a].

Rhinitis among bakers is common and usually precedes asthma. Conjunctivitis and skin symptoms may also occur. Atopy is a risk factor, but gender, age, and smoking habits do not have a significant influence on sensitization or disease [De Zotti et al. 1994; Baur et al. 1998; Houba et al. 1998b]. Symptoms develop after a latency period of months or years, even decades, and risk increases with increased exposure concentration. In addition to allergy, non-specific mucous membrane and respiratory irritation also occur frequently among bakers, possibly more commonly than allergic symptoms [Houba et al. 1998a].

Wheat and other cereal flours are the main causes of baker's allergy. Wheat flour is a complex mixture that contains at least 40 antigens [Houba et al. 1996]. Other common allergens in bakeries are the enzymatic dough improvers, of which fungal α-amylase is the most frequently reported cause of allergy. Epidemiologic studies have demonstrated prevalences of sensitization of 5%–28% to wheat and 2%–16% to α-amylase [Houba et al. 1996]. Variability in these prevalences is due to use of different methodologies for measuring sensitization between studies. The prevalence of sensitization to BAA, allergy, and asthma among bakers in the U.S. is unknown, as is the range of exposures encountered in U.S. bakeries.

Background sensitization is also found in the general population. A study of 416 animal laboratory employees documented that 1.7% had positive skin prick tests to fungal α-amylase and 2.1% to wheat [Houba et al. 1996]. One study demonstrated sensitization prevalences to wheat of 1.2% for animal health apprentices and 4.1% for dental hygiene apprentices [Gautrin et al. 1997]. A NIOSH study of 534 blood donors demonstrated the prevalence of specific IgE to wheat (3.6%), flour (5.8%), and α-amylase (1.0%) [Biagini et al. 2004].

Baker's Dermatitis

The bakery employee's skin is exposed to wet dough, flours with additives, spices, water, and detergents. This exposure can cause contact allergy and/or irritation of the skin, and bakers have an increased risk of hand eczema [Brisman et al. 1998; Vein 2000]. Work-related contact urticaria and protein dermatitis have also been reported [Odom and Maibach 1976; Morren et al. 1993; Kanerva et al. 1996].

References

ACGIH [2007]. 2007 TLVs® and BEIs®: threshold limit values for chemical substances and physical agents and biological exposure indices. Cincinnati, OH: American Conference of Governmental Industrial Hygienists.

AIHA [2007]. 2007 Emergency response planning guidelines (ERPG) & workplace environmental exposure levels (WEEL) handbook. Fairfax, VA: American Industrial Hygiene Association.

Baur X, Degens P, Sander I [1998]. Baker's asthma: still among the most frequent occupational respiratory disorders. J All Clin Immunol 102(6 Pt 1):984–997.

Biagini RE, MacKenzie BA, Sammons DL, Smith JP, Striley CA, Robertson SK, Snawder JE [2004]. Evaluation of the prevalence of anti-wheat, anti-flour dust, and anti-α-amylase specific IgE antibodies in US blood donors. Ann Allergy Asthma Immun 92(6):649–653.

Brisman J, Meding B, Jarvholm B [1998]. Occurrence of self reported hand eczema in Swedish bakers. Occup Environ Med 55(11):750–754.

Brisman J [2002]. Baker's asthma. Occup Environ Med 59(7):498–502.

CFR. Code of Federal Regulations. Washington, DC: U.S. Government Printing Office, Office of the Federal Register.

De Zotti R, Larese F, Bovenzi M, Negro C, Molinari S [1994]. Allergic airway disease in Italian bakers and pastry makers. Occup Environ Med 51(8):548–552.

Gautrin D, Infante-Rivard C, Dao TV, Magnan-Larose M, Desjardins J, Malo JM [1997]. Specific IgE-dependent sensitization, atopy, and bronchial hyperresponsiveness in apprentices starting exposure to protein derived agents. Am J Respir Crit Care Med 155(6):1841–1847.

Houba R, Heederick D, Doekes G, van Run P [1996]. Exposure sensitization relationship for α-amylase allergens in the baking industry. Am J Respir Crit Care Med 154(1):130–136.

Houba R, Doekes G, Heederick D [1998a]. Occupational respiratory allergy in bakery workers: a review of the literature. Am J Ind Med 34(6):529–546.

Houba R, Heederik D, Doekes G [1998b]. Wheat sensitization and work related symptoms in the baking industry are preventable: an epidemiologic study. Am J Respir Crit Care Med 158(5 Pt 1):1499–1503.

Kanerva L, Toikkanen J, Jolanki R, Estlander T [1996]. Statistical data on occupational contact urticaria. Contact Dermatitis 35(4):229–233.

Morren M, Janssens V, Dooms-Goossens A [1993]. alpha-Amylase, a flour additive: an important cause of protein contact dermatitis in bakers. J Am Acad Dermatol 29(5 Pt 1):723–728.

NIOSH [2005]. NIOSH pocket guide to chemical hazards. Cincinnati, OH: U.S. Department of Health and Human Services, Centers for Disease Control and Prevention, National Institute for Occupational Safety and Health, DHHS (NIOSH) Publication No. 2005-149. [www.cdc.gov/niosh/npg/]. Date accessed: Janaury 2009.

Odom RB, Maibach H [1976]. Contact urticaria: a different contact dermatitis. Cutis 18(5):672–676.

Vein NK [2000]. Bakers. In: Kanerva L, Wilsner P, Wahlberg JE, Maibach HI, eds. Handbook of occupational dermatology. Berlin: Springer-Verlag. pp. 817-821.

Study Population

The study population included all employees at the Sara Lee Bakery in Sacramento, California. All employees were asked to participate in order to compare sensitization and symptom prevalences between groups of employees with differing levels of exposure to bakery antigens, and to most accurately characterize exposure in the different departments of the bakery.

Informed Consent and Notification

All potential study participants were given a consent form to read and sign should they wish to participate in the study. Each study participant was informed in writing of the results of his or her serum tests and what they meant.

Biological Samples

Approximately 15 mL of whole blood were collected from each of the participants who consented to have blood drawn. Venipuncture was performed by trained technicians following the universal precautions for working with blood and blood products specified by CDC and OSHA [CDC 1998; 29 CFR 1910.1000]. After venipuncture, the blood was centrifuged and the serum transported to the NIOSH laboratory for analysis. Serum was tested for total IgE; IgE specific to flour, wheat, and α-amylase; and for a variety of common aeroallergens to assess atopy.

Specific IgE was measured using an IMMULITE® 2000 3gAllergy™ instrument (DPC, Los Angeles, California). The IMMULITE 2000 is an FDA-cleared enzyme-enhanced chemiluminescent enzyme immunoassay that quantifies specific IgE antibody. Briefly, a streptavidin-coated bead, biotinylated liquid allergen, and serum sample are incubated for 30 minutes. After a spin wash, an alkaline phosphatase labeled monoclonal antibody specific for human IgE is added and another 30-minute incubation follows. The bead is washed again, and the enzyme label is measured with a chemiluminescent substrate (phosphate ester of adamantyl dioxetane). Specific IgE was measured against the following allergens: fungal α-amylase (K87M), flour (K301M), and wheat (F4M). Specific IgE calibrators and positive controls are included with the kit. A negative serum control (human serum with no detectable allergen-specific IgE) and an internal positive quality control serum sample (serum positive to Dermatophagoides farinae), recommended by the manufacturer, is also run in all assays.

The IMMULITE 2000 has an FDA-cleared cutoff of 0.10 kU/L IgE. The insert for the IMMULITE 3gAllergy Specific IgE Universal Kit describes two scoring systems, both of which classify specific IgE levels ≥ 0.10 kU/L–0.34 kU/L (standard classification) and ≥ 0.11 kU/L–0.24 kU/L (extended classification) as very low. Traditionally, a level ≥ 0.35 kU/L is considered Class 1, or positive.

AlaTOP was measured using the IMMULITE 2000 AlaTOP Allergy Screen for 12 allergens. This method is a FDA-cleared qualitative chemiluminescent enzyme-labeled sequential immunoassay, based on liquid ligand-labeled allergens, monoclonal antibodies, and separation by anti-ligand coated solid phase. The allergens are covalently bound to a soluble polymer/copolymer matrix, which in turn is labeled with a ligand; anti-ligand is coated on the polystyrene bead to capture the ligand-labeled allergens. The 12 allergens included on the matrix are Dermatophagoides pteronyssinus (dust mite), cat epithelium, dog dander, Cynodon dactylon (Bermuda grass), Phleum pretense (timothy grass), Penicillium notatum, Alternaria tenuis, Ambrosia artemisiifolia (common ragweed), Plantago lanceolata (English plantain), Parietaria officinalis (wall pelitory), Betula papyrifera (paper birch), and Cryptomeria japonica (Japanese cedar). A positive and negative reference serum is included in each assay. A reactive result indicates that antibodies to one or more of the component allergens in the panel are present in the patient sample, and that patient is classified as atopic. A non-reactive result indicates non-detectable antibodies to the component allergens.

Total IgE was measured using the IMMULITE© 2000 Total IgE. This method is an FDA-cleared solid phase, chemiluminescent immunometric assay using the same technology as outlined above. IgE levels normally show a slow increase during childhood, reaching adult levels in the second decade of life. In general, the total IgE level increases with the number of allergies a person has and with the amount of exposure to relevant allergens. Other investigators studying baker's asthma have defined atopy as a total serum IgE above 100 kU/L [Suarthana et al. 2005].

Questionnaire

All participants in this evaluation completed a questionnaire. Its questions concerned demographics (age, sex, job title, years worked, work department); personal history of allergies, eczema, asthma, and smoking; having upper and lower respiratory symptoms at work in the last month (unrelated to a cold or respiratory infection); and whether those symptoms got better on days off work. Symptoms were considered work related if they were present at work and improved on days away from work. Participants were classified as current, former, or never smokers.

Industrial Hygiene

PBZ and GA air sampling was conducted to characterize employees' overall exposures to BAA. Full shift PBZ and GA air measurements for inhalable flour dust and total dust were collected in the bread and bun production, distribution, engineering, and sanitation departments; and the office and plant management areas. While both PBZ and GA samples were taken in multiple work areas, GA samples were primarily taken in areas where exposure was thought to be low (i.e., office areas). No measurements were taken for transportation workers because they do not work in the bakery building, but drive trucks to deliver product to retailers.

Total dust samples were analyzed by the NIOSH contract lab for weight gain following NIOSH Method 500 [NIOSH 2008]. The total dust samples had a limit of detection that ranged from 46 to 100 micrograms and a limit of quantitation that ranged from 150 to 220 micrograms, depending on the batch.

Inhalable flour dust samples were collected using IOM samplers with Teflon® filters (pore size 1.0 micron with laminated polytetrafluoroethylene support). Total dust samples were collected using closed-face 37-millimeter cassettes with polyvinyl chloride filters (pore size 5.0 microns). Samples were connected to personal sampling pumps calibrated to a flow rate of 2 liters per minute. Both IOM and 37-millimeter cassettes were changed throughout the shift to prevent overloading the sampling media.

Inhalable flour dust samples were stored at ambient temperatures in sealed containers to prevent additional exposure to moisture during storage and shipment. A recording high-low thermometer was added to all shipping containers to record maximal temperature transients of the samples. The samples were first analyzed by the NIOSH contract lab for inhalable flour dust (weight gain). The flour dust samples had a limit of detection that ranged from 46 to 100 micrograms and a limit of quantitation that ranged from 150 to 350 micrograms, depending on the batch.

Following the weight gain analysis, the inhalable flour dust samples were then shipped to the Institute for Risk Assessment Sciences, University of Utrecht, Utrecht, Netherlands, where they were analyzed using the methods outlined below for α-amylase and wheat allergens.

Wheat allergens were recovered from the filters by extraction with 2 5 mL 0.15 M phosphate-buffered saline (pH 7.4), and concentrations were measured in the extract by inhibition immunoassay, using a pool of human immunoglobulin G4 polyclonal antibodies. The limit of detection for this method was 50 nanograms per milliliter [Hauba et al. 1996]. The α-amylase allergens were measured using a sandwich enzyme immunoassay with affinity-purified polyclonal rabbit IgG antibodies. The limit of detection for this method was 100 picograms per milliliter [Hauba et al. 1997].

Statistical Analysis

SAS Version 9.1.3 software (SAS Institute, Cary, North Carolina) and StatXact Version 6 software (Cytel Software Corporation, Cambridge, MA) were used for the statistical analyses. Results with p values ≤ 0.05 were considered statistically significant. Geometric means and medians are reported for environmental samples because some distributions were lognormal and others were not. PRs were used to compare the prevalence of symptoms and the prevalence of sensitization to BAA between exposure groups. A PR greater than 1 indicates a positive relationship between a having a symptom/sensitization and being in the higher-exposure group. Along with the PR, a 95% CI for the PR was calculated. The PR is considered statistically significant if the 95% CI does not include the number 1. Chi square or Fisher's exact tests were also used to compare the prevalence of sensitization to BAA between atopics and non-atopics, and the prevalence of self-reported, work-related symptoms among employees who are sensitized to flour dust, α-amylase, or wheat and those who are not. Total IgE was log normally distributed so we transformed the data, and used the Student's t-test to determine any difference between exposure groups. Pearson's correlation coefficient was used to determine the correlation between the log-transformed total dust and inhalable flour dust concentrations, as well as between the log-transformed α-amylase and inhalable flour dust concentrations, and the log-transformed wheat and inhalable flour dust concentrations.

Statistical analysis of air sampling results included the use of imputed concentrations where the sample results were less than the limit of detection. For samples that were less than the limit of detection (i.e., ND), a concentration was calculated by dividing the reported limit of detection by the square root of 2 and then by the individual sample volume [Hornung et al. 1990]. For samples between the limit of detection and limit of quantitation (i.e., trace), a concentration was calculated by dividing the estimated laboratory result by the individual sample volume. Concentrations for samples above the limit of quantitation were calculated by dividing the reported laboratory result by the individual sample volume. In this report values less than the limit of quantitation are reported either as ND or trace, not as the calculated concentration used in the statistical analysis.

Air sampling measures are reported using a modified significant figure convention. Individual measures are reported to 2 significant figures and GM and median are reported to an additional figure. The use of exponential notation has not been followed.

References

CDC [1998]. Guideline for infection control in health care personnel. Am J Infec Control 26: 289-354.

CFR. Code of Federal Regulations. Washington, DC: U.S. Government Printing Office, Office of the Federal Register.

Hornung RW, Reed LD [1990]. Estimation of average concentration in the presence of nondetectable values. Appl Occup Environ Hyg 5(1):46-51.

Houba R, van Run P, Heederik D, Doekes G [1996]. Wheat antigen exposure assessment for epidemiological studies in bakeries using personal dust sampling and inhibition ELISA. Clin Exp Allergy 26(2):154-163.

Houba R, van Run P, Doekes G, Heederik D, Spithoven J [1997]. Airborne levels of alpha amylase allergens in bakeries. J Allergy Clin Immunol 99(3):286-292.

NIOSH [2008]. NIOSH manual of analytical methods (NMAM®). 4th ed. Schlecht PC, O'Connor PF, eds. Cincinnati, OH: U.S. Department of Health and Human Services, Centers for Disease Control and Prevention, National Institute for Occupational Safety and Health, DHHS (NIOSH) Publication 94-113 (August, 1994); 1st Supplement Publication 96-135, 2nd Supplement Publication 98-119; 3rd Supplement 2003-154. [www.cdc.gov/niosh/nmam/]. Date accessed: January 2009.

Suarthana E, Vergouwe Y, Nieuwenhuijsen M, Heederik D, Grobbee DE, Meijer E [2005]. Diagnostic model for sensitization in workers exposed to occupational high molecular weight allergens. Am J Ind Med 48(3):168-174.

Individual air sample results

Department	Job title	Inhalable flour dust (mg/m^3)	Total dust (mg/m^3)	α-amylase (ng/m^3)	Wheat (ng/m^3)
Bread production	Divider[†]	1.3**	1.3	¶	6,700
	Divider	6.3**	‡	0.45	89,000
	Divider	3.0**	0.79	0.43	15,000
	Divider	3.7**	‡	¶	16,000
	Foreperson	4.5**	‡	220	36,000
	Foreperson	4.5**	‡	32	32,000
	Foreperson	2.6**	‡	20	9,500
	Foreperson	7.3**	2.4	4.9	19,000
	Mixer[†]	8.3**	3.5	3.2	33,000
	Mixer	18**	30[††, ‡‡]	440	69,000
	Mixer	3.8**	3.4	480	24,000
	Mixer	1.5**	2.0	890	2,900
	Moulder[†]	§	§	¶	¶
	Moulder	4.0**	1.9	1.2	40,000
	Moulder	2.4**	‡	0.77	19,000
	Oven	§	‡	¶	1,500
	Oven	0.50**	§	¶	2,200
	Oven	0.55**	‡	¶	780
	Scaler	20**	5.1[‡‡]	4.2	13,000
	Scaler	7.8**	‡	2.0	10,000
	Scaler[†]	1.1**	‡	4.1	6,700
	Sponge mixer	27**	28[††, ‡‡]	1,200	150,000
	Sponge mixer	65**	‡	61	180,000
	Sponge mixer	8.2**	‡	4.4	25,000
	Sponge mixer	28**	25[††, ‡‡]	9.1	100,000
	Utility	0.84**	‡	0.55	5,700
	Wrap[†]	§	§	¶	¶
	Wrap	§	‡	¶	¶
	Wrap	0.86**	‡	¶	1,900
	Wrap	0.69**	‡	¶	2,600
	Wrap	1.4**	‡	¶	1,900
	Wrap	§	‡	¶	¶
	Wrap	0.48	‡	¶	¶
	Wrap	§	‡	¶	¶
Bun production	*	18**	4.8[‡‡]	17	58,000
	Divider	5.5**	‡	0.30	15,000
	Divider	2.3**	‡	¶	19,000
	Divider	3.4**	‡	0.40	31,000
	Foreperson	2.0**	1.6	2.1	12,000
	Foreperson	3.4**	‡	1.1	26,000
	Jober	1.2**	‡	¶	2,900
	Mixer	2.7**	‡	12	13,000
	Mixer	2.6**	‡	11,000	10,000
	Mixer[†]	1.3**	1.2	20	6,100
	Mixer	8.5**	‡	34	38,000

Individual air sample results (continued)

Department	Job title	Inhalable flour dust (mg/m^3)	Total dust (mg/m^3)	α-amylase (ng/m^3)	Wheat (ng/m^3)
Bun production (continued)	Moulder	7.3**	‡	1.2	150,000
	Oven	0.24	‡	0.069	1,600
	Pan line	12**	‡	1.1	320,000
	Pan line	8.8**	7.4‡‡	9.0	62,000
	Pan line	3.7**	‡	1.1	20,000
	Pan line†	2.6**	1.5	3.7	29,000
	Pan line	0.45	‡	¶	900
	Pan stacker	1.2**	‡	¶	3,600
	Wrap	§	‡	¶	¶
	Wrap†	0.49**	¶	¶	950
	Wrap†	¶	¶	¶	¶
	Wrap	§	‡	¶	¶
	Wrap	§	§	¶	¶
	Wrap†	§	¶	¶	280
	Wrap	§	‡	¶	¶
	Wrap	§	‡	¶	2,000
	Wrap	§	‡	¶	690
	Wrap	§	‡	¶	¶
	Wrap	§	‡	¶	¶
	Wrap	§	§	¶	¶
	Wrap	0.79**	§	¶	¶
	Wrap†	‡	§	‡	‡
Distribution	*, †	¶	¶	¶	¶
	*, †	§	¶	¶	¶
	*, †	¶	‡	¶	¶
	*, †	¶	¶	¶	¶
	Foreperson	¶	‡	¶	¶
	*, †	¶	‡	¶	¶
Engineering	*	0.62**	‡	¶	1,800
	*	0.42**	§	¶	¶
	*	2.4**	§	0.27	28,000
	*	0.78**	§	¶	2,200
	*	0.43	§	¶	330
	*	§	§	¶	280
Office and plant management	*, †	¶	¶	¶	¶
	*, †	¶	‡	¶	¶
	*, †	¶	‡	1.1	¶
	*, †	¶	¶	¶	¶
Sanitation	*	0.77**	‡	0.20	4,500
	*	0.68**	‡	25	2,700
	*	21**	‡	5.4	150,000
	*	0.81**	‡	¶	1,300
	*	64**	‡	10	900,000
	*	0.55**	§	¶	1,700
	*	1.0**	0.76	¶	6,300

Individual air sample results (continued)

Department	Job title	Inhalable flour dust (mg/m^3)	Total dust (mg/m^3)	α-amylase (ng/m^3)	Wheat (ng/m^3)
Sanitation (continued)	*	1.5**	‡	¶	7,800
	*	0.70**	‡	¶	3,400
	*	21**	‡	3.0	130,000
	*	1.8**	‡	1.8	1,900
	*	1.4**	‡	21	4,400
	*	1.0**	‡	¶	2,700
	*	1.1**	‡	4.3	4,600
	*	2.8**	‡	0.18	12,000
	*	3.3**	‡	¶	8,300
	*	5.4**	‡	2.8	17,000
	*	25**	‡	31	170,000
	*	0.94**	‡	¶	4,100
	Foreperson	4.4**	‡	16	30,000

*No specific job title provided

[†]General area sample

[‡]No sample collected

[§]Trace: between 0.12 and 0.42 mg/m^3 for inhalable flour dust, and 0.077 and 0.25 mg/m^3 for total dust (based on an average sample volume)

[¶]ND: < 0.12 mg/m^3 for inhalable flour dust, <0.18 ng/m^3 for α-amylase, < 300 ng/m^3 for wheat, and < 0.077 ng/m^3 for total dust (based on an average sample volume)

**Exceeds the CalOSHA PEL for inhalable flour dust of 0.5 mg/m^3

[††]Exceeds the OSHA PEL for particulates not otherwise regulated of 15 mg/m^3

[‡‡]Exceeds the NIOSH PEL for grain dust (oat, wheat, and barley) of 4 mg/m^3

ACKNOWLEDGMENTS AND AVAILABILITY OF REPORT

The Hazard Evaluations and Technical Assistance Branch (HETAB) of the National Institute for Occupational Safety and Health (NIOSH) conducts field investigations of possible health hazards in the workplace. These investigations are conducted under the authority of Section 20(a)(6) of the Occupational Safety and Health (OSHA) Act of 1970, 29 U.S.C. 669(a)(6) which authorizes the Secretary of Health and Human Services, following a written request from any employer or authorized representative of employees, to determine whether any substance normally found in the place of employment has potentially toxic effects in such concentrations as used or found. HETAB also provides, upon request, technical and consultative assistance to federal, state, and local agencies; labor; industry; and other groups or individuals to control occupational health hazards and to prevent related trauma and disease.

The findings and conclusions in this report are those of the authors and do not necessarily represent the views of NIOSH. Mention of any company or product does not constitute endorsement by NIOSH. In addition, citations to Web sites external to NIOSH do not constitute NIOSH endorsement of the sponsoring organizations or their programs or products. Furthermore, NIOSH is not responsible for the content of these Web sites. All Web addresses referenced in this document were accessible as of the publication date.

This report was prepared by Elena H. Page, Chad H. Dowell, and Charles A. Mueller of HETAB, Division of Surveillance, Hazard Evaluations and Field Studies (DSHEFS), and Raymond E. Biagini of the Division of Applied Research and Technology (DART). Industrial hygiene field assistance was provided by Gregory Burr, Kevin L. Dunn, and Bradley King, DSHEFS, and Duane Hammond of DART. Medical field assistance was provided by Barbara MacKenzie, Deborah Sammons, Christine Toennis, and John Snawder of DART. Analytical support was provided by Barbara MacKenzie of DART; DataChem Laboratories, Clayton Group Services, and the Universiteit Utrecht Institute for Risk Assessment Sciences. Editorial assistance was provided by Ellen Galloway. Health communication assistance was provided by Stefanie Evans. Desktop publishing was performed by Robin Smith.

Copies of this report have been sent to employee and management representatives at the Sara Lee Bakery and the OSHA Regional Office. This report is not copyrighted and may be freely reproduced. The report may be viewed and printed from the following internet address: www.cdc.gov/niosh/hhe. Copies may be purchased from the National Technical Information Service (NTIS) at 5825 Port Royal Road, Springfield, Virginia 22161.